Table of Contents

Arthritis means joint inflammation, but the term is used to describe around 200 conditions that affect joints, the tissues that surround the joint, and other connective tissue. It is a rheumatic condition.

The most common form of arthritis is osteoarthritis. Other common rheumatic conditions related to arthritis include Trusted Source gout, fibromyalgia, and rheumatoid arthritis (RA).

Rheumatic conditions tend to involve pain, aching, stiffness, and swelling in and around one or more joints. The symptoms can develop gradually or suddenly. Certain rheumatic conditions can also involve Trusted Source the immune system and various internal organs of the body.

Some forms of arthritis, such as rheumatoid arthritis and lupus (SLE), can affect multiple organs and cause widespread symptoms.

According to the Centers for Disease Control and Prevention (CDC), 54.4 million Trusted Source adults in the United States have received a diagnosis of some form of arthritis. Of these, 23.7 million people have their activity curtailed in some way by their condition.

Arthritis is more common among adults aged 65 years or older, but it can affect people of all ages, including children.

Fast facts on arthritis

Here are some key points about arthritis. More detail is in the main article.

• Arthritis refers to around 200 rheumatic diseases and conditions that affect joints, including lupus and rheumatoid arthritis.

• It can cause a range of symptoms and impair a person's ability to perform everyday tasks.

• Physical activity has a positive effect on arthritis and can improve pain, function, and mental health.

• Factors in the development of arthritis include injury, abnormal metabolism, genetic makeup, infections, and immune system dysfunction.

• Treatment aims to control pain, minimize joint damage, and improve or maintain quality of life. It involves medications, physical therapies, and patient education and support.

Treatment
The doctor will likely recommend a course of physical therapies to help you manage some of the symptoms of arthritis.

Treatment for arthritis aims to control pain, minimize joint damage, and improve or maintain function and quality of life.

A range of medications and lifestyle strategies can help achieve this and protect joints from further damage.

Treatment might involve Trusted Source:

• medications

• non-pharmacologic therapies

• physical or occupational therapy

• splints or joint assistive aids

• patient education and support

• weight loss

• surgery, including joint replacement

Medication

Non-inflammatory types of arthritis, such as osteoarthritis, are often treated with pain-reducing medications, physical activity, weight loss if the person is overweight, and self-management education.

These treatments are also applied to inflammatory types of arthritis, such as RA, along with anti-inflammatory medications such as corticosteroids and non-steroidal anti-inflammatory drugs (NSAIDs), disease-modifying anti-rheumatic drugs (DMARDs), and a relatively new class of drugs known as biologics.

Medications will depend on the type of arthritis. Commonly used drugs include:

• Analgesics: these reduce pain, but have no effect on inflammation. Examples include acetaminophen (Tylenol), tramadol (Ultram) and narcotics containing oxycodone (Percocet, Oxycontin) or hydrocodone (Vicodin, Lortab). Tylenol is available to purchase online.

• Non-steroidal anti-inflammatory drugs (NSAIDs): these reduce both pain and inflammation. NSAIDs include available to purchase over-the-counter or online, includeing ibuprofen (Advil, Motrin IB) and naproxen sodium (Aleve). Some NSAIDs are available as creams, gels or patches which can be applied to specific joints.

• Counterirritants: some creams and ointments contain menthol or capsaicin, the ingredient that makes hot peppers spicy. Rubbing these on the skin over a painful joint can modulate pain signals from the joint and lessen pain. Various creams are available to purchase online.

• Disease-modifying antirheumatic drugs (DMARDs): used to treat RA, DMARDs slow or stop the immune system from attacking the joints. Examples include methotrexate (Trexall) and hydroxychloroquine (Plaquenil).

• Biologics: used with DMARDs, biologic response modifiers are genetically engineered drugs that target various protein molecules involved in the immune response. Examples include etanercept (Enbrel) and infliximab (Remicade).

• Corticosteroids: prednisone and cortisone reduce inflammation and suppress the immune system.

Causes

There is no single cause of all types of arthritis. The cause or causes vary according to the type or form of arthritis.

Possible causes may include:

• injury, leading to degenerative arthritis

- abnormal metabolism, leading to gout and pseudogout

- inheritance, such as in osteoarthritis

- infections, such as in the arthritis of Lyme disease

- immune system dysfunction, such as in RA and SLE

Most types of arthritis are linked to a combination of factors, but some have no obvious cause and appear to be unpredictable in their emergence.

Some people may be genetically more likely to develop certain arthritic conditions. Additional factors, such as previous injury, infection, smoking and physically demanding occupations, can interact with genes to further increase the risk of arthritis.

Diet and nutrition can play a role in managing arthritis and the risk of arthritis, although specific foods, food sensitivities or intolerances are not known to cause arthritis.

Foods that increase inflammation, particularly animal-derived foods and diets high in refined sugar, can make symptoms worse, as can eating foods that provoke an immune system response.

Gout is one type of arthritis that is closely linked to diet, as it is caused by elevated levels of uric acid which can be a result of a diet high in purines.

Diets that contain high-purine foods, such as seafood, red wine, and meats, can trigger a gout flare-up. Vegetables and other plant foods that contain high levels of purines do not appear to exacerbate gout symptoms, however.

Certain risk factors have been associated with arthritis. Some of these are modifiable while others are not.

Non-modifiable arthritis risk factors:

• Age: the risk of developing most types of arthritis increases with age.

• Sex: most types of arthritis are more common in females, and 60 percent of all people with arthritis are female. Gout is more common in males than females.

• Genetic factors: specific genes are associated with a higher risk of certain types of arthritis, such as rheumatoid arthritis (RA), systemic lupus erythematosus (SLE) and ankylosing spondylitis.

Modifiable arthritis risk factors:

• Overweight and obesity: excess weight can contribute to both the onset and progression of knee osteoarthritis.

• Joint injuries: damage to a joint can contribute to the development of osteoarthritis in that joint.

• Infection: many microbial agents can infect joints and trigger the development of various forms of arthritis.

• Occupation: certain occupations that involve repetitive knee bending and squatting are associated with osteoarthritis of the knee.

Comorbidities

More than half of adults in the U.S. with arthritis report high blood pressure. High blood pressure is associated with heart disease, the most common comorbidity among adults with arthritis.

Around 1 in 5 of adults in the U.S. who have arthritis are smokers. Smoking is associated with chronic respiratory conditions, the second most common comorbidity among adults with arthritis.

Types

There are around 200 types of arthritis, or musculoskeletal conditions. These are split into seven main groups:

1. Inflammatory arthritis

2. Degenerative or mechanical arthritis

3. Soft tissue musculoskeletal pain

4. Back pain

5. Connective tissue disease

6. Infectious arthritis

7. Metabolic arthritis.

Inflammatory arthritis

Inflammation is a normal part of the body's healing process. The inflammation tends to occur as a defense against viruses and bacteria or as a response to injuries such as burns. However, with inflammatory arthritis, inflammation occurs in people for no apparent reason.

Inflammatory arthritis can affect several joints, damaging the surface of the joints and the underlying bone.

Inflammatory arthritis is characterized by damaging inflammation that does not occur as a normal reaction to injury or infection. This type of inflammation is unhelpful and instead causes damage in the affected joints, resulting in pain, stiffness and swelling.

Inflammatory arthritis can affect several joints, and the inflammation can damage the surface of the joints and also the underlying bone.

Examples of inflammatory arthritis include:

• Rheumatoid arthritis (RA)

• Reactive arthritis

• Ankylosing spondylitis

• Arthritis associated with colitis or psoriasis

The word "arthritis" means "joint inflammation," but inflammation may also affect the tendons and ligaments surrounding the joint.

Degenerative or mechanical arthritis

Degenerative or mechanical arthritis refers to a group of conditions that mainly involve damage to the cartilage that covers the ends of the bones.

The main job of the smooth, slippery cartilage is to help the joints glide and move smoothly. This type of arthritis causes the cartilage to become thinner and rougher.

To compensate for the loss of cartilage and changes in joint function, the body begins to remodel the bone in an attempt to restore stability. This can cause undesirable bony growths to develop, called osteophytes. The joint can become misshapen. This condition is commonly called osteoarthritis.

Osteoarthritis can also result from previous damage to the joint such as a fracture or previous inflammation in the joint.

Soft tissue musculoskeletal pain

Soft tissue musculoskeletal pain is felt in tissues other than the joints and bones. The pain often affects a part of the body following injury or overuse, such as tennis elbow, and originates from the muscles or soft tissues supporting the joints.

Pain that is more widespread and associated with other symptoms may indicate fibromyalgia.

Back pain

Back pain can arise from the muscles, discs, nerves, ligaments, bones, or joints. Back pain may stem from problems with organs inside the body. It can also be a result of referred pain, for example, when a problem elsewhere in the body leads to pain in the back.

There may be a specific cause, such as osteoarthritis. This is often called spondylosis when it occurs in the spine. Imaging tests or a physical examination may detect this.

A "slipped" disc is another cause of back pain, as is osteoporosis, or thinning of the bones.

If a doctor cannot identify the exact cause of back pain, it is often described as "non-specific" pain.

Connective tissue disease (CTD)

Connective tissues support, bind together, or separate other body tissues and organs. They include tendons, ligaments, and cartilage.

CTD involves joint pain and inflammation. The inflammation may also occur in other tissues, including the skin, muscles, lungs, and kidneys. This can result in various symptoms besides painful joints, and it may require consultation with a number of different specialists.

Examples of CTD include:

• SLE, or lupus

• scleroderma, or systemic sclerosis

• dermatomyositis.

Infectious arthritis

A bacterium, virus, or fungus that enters a joint can sometimes cause inflammation.

Organisms that can infect joints include:

• Salmonella and Shigella, spread through food poisoning or contamination

• chlamydia and gonorrhea, which are sexually transmitted diseases (STDs)

• hepatitis C, a blood-to-blood infection that may be spread through shared needles or transfusions

A joint infection can often be cleared with antibiotics or other antimicrobial medication. However, the arthritis can sometimes become chronic, and joint damage may be irreversible if the infection has persisted for some time.

Metabolic arthritis

Uric acid is a chemical created when the body breaks down substances called purines. Purines are found in human cells and several foods.

Most uric acid dissolves in blood and travels to the kidneys. From there, it passes out in urine. Some people have high levels of uric, acid because they either naturally produce more than they need or their body cannot clear the uric acid quickly enough.

Uric acid builds up and accumulates in some people and forms needle-like crystals in the joint, resulting in sudden spikes of extreme joint pain or a gout attack.

Gout can either come and go in episodes or become chronic if uric acid levels are not reduced.

It commonly affects a single joint or a small number of joints, such as the big toe and hands. It usually affects the extremities. One theory is that uric acid crystals form in cooler joints, away from the main warmth of the body.

Some of the more common types of arthritis are discussed below.

Rheumatoid arthritis

Rheumatoid arthritis and osteoarthritis share some characteristics, but they are different conditions.

Rheumatoid arthritis (RA) occurs when the body's immune system attacks the tissues of the body, specifically connective tissue, leading to joint inflammation, pain, and degeneration of the joint tissue.

Cartilage is a flexible, connective tissue in joints that absorb the pressure and shock created by movement like running and walking. It also protects the joints and allows for smooth movement.

Persistent inflammation in the synovia leads to the degeneration of cartilage and bone. This can then lead to joint deformity, pain, swelling, and redness.

RA can appear at any age and is associated with fatigue and prolonged stiffness after rest.

RA causes premature mortalityTrusted Source and disability and it can compromise quality of life. Conditions it is linked to include cardiovascular diseases, such as ischemic heart disease and stroke.

Diagnosing RA early gives a better chance of learning how to manage symptoms successfully. This can reduce the impact of the disease on quality of life.

Osteoarthritis

Osteoarthritis is caused by a reduction in the normal amount of cartilage tissue through wear and tear throughout life.

Osteoarthritis is a common degenerative joint disease that affects the cartilage Trusted Source, joint lining and ligaments, and underlying bone of a joint.

The breakdown of these tissues eventually leads to pain and joint stiffness.

The joints most often affected by osteoarthritis are those that get heavy use, such as hips, knees, hands, the spine, the base of the thumb, and the big toe joint.

Childhood arthritis

This can refer to a number of types of arthritis. Juvenile idiopathic arthritis (JIA), also known as juvenile rheumatoid arthritis (JRA), is the most common Trusted Source type.

Arthritis in childhood can cause permanent damage to joints, and there is no cure. However, remission is possible, during which time the disease remains inactive.

It may be due to immune system problems.

Septic arthritis

This is thought to affect between 2 and 10 people in every 100,000 in the general population. Among people with RA, it may affect 30 to 70 people per 100,000.

Septic arthritis is a joint inflammation that results from a bacterial or fungal infection. It commonly affects the knee and hip.

It can develop when bacteria or other disease-causing micro-organisms spread through the blood to a joint, or when the joint is directly infected with a microorganism through injury or surgery.

Bacteria such as Staphylococcus, Streptococcus, or Neisseria gonorrhoeae cause most cases of acute septic arthritis. Organisms such as Mycobacterium tuberculosis and Candida albicans cause chronic septic arthritis. This is less common than acute septic arthritis.

Septic arthritis may occur at any age. In infants, it may occur before the age of 3 years. The hip is a common site of infection at this age.

Septic arthritis is uncommon from 3 years to adolescence. Children with septic arthritis are more likely than adults to be infected with Group B Streptococcus or Haemophilus influenzae if they have not been vaccinated.

The incidence of bacterial arthritis caused by infection with H. influenzae has decreased by around 70 percent to 80 percent since the use of the H. influenzae b (Hib) vaccine became common.

The following conditions increase the risk of developing septic arthritis:

- existing joint disease or damage

- artificial joint implants

- bacterial infection elsewhere in the body

- presence of bacteria in the blood

- chronic illness or disease (such as diabetes, RA and sickle cell disease)

- intravenous (IV) or injection drug use

- medications that suppress the immune system

- recent joint injury

- recent joint arthroscopy or other surgery

- conditions such as HIV, that weaken immunity

- diabetes

• older age

Septic arthritis is a rheumatologic emergency as it can lead to rapid joint destruction. It can be fatal.

Fibromyalgia

Fibromyalgia affects an estimated 4 million Trusted Source adults in the U.S, or around 2 percent of the population.

It usually starts during middle age or after, but it can affect children.

Fibromyalgia can involve:

• widespread pain

• sleep disturbance

• fatigue

• depression

• problems with thinking and remembering

The person may experience abnormal pain processing, where they reacts strongly to something that other people would not find painful.

There may also be tingling or numbness in the hands and feet, pain in the jaw, and digestive problems.

The causes of fibromyalgia are unknown, but some factors have been loosely associated with disease onset:

• stressful or traumatic events

• post-traumatic stress disorder (PTSD)

• injuries due to repetitive movements

• illness, for example viral infections

• having lupus, RA, or chronic fatigue syndrome

• family history

• obesity

It is more common among females.

Psoriatic arthritis

Psoriatic arthritis is a joint problem that often occurs with a skin condition called psoriasis. It is thought to affect between 0.3 and 1 percent of the population in the U.S., and between 6 and 42 percent of people with psoriasis.

Most people who have psoriatic arthritis and psoriasis develop psoriasis first and then psoriatic arthritis, but joint problems can occasionally occur before skin lesions appear.

The exact cause of psoriatic arthritis is not known, but it appears to involve the immune system attacking healthy cells and tissue. The abnormal immune response causes inflammation in the joints and an overproduction of skin cells. Damage to the joints can result.

Factors that increase the risk, include:
• having psoriasis

• family history

• being aged from 30 to 50 year

People with psoriatic arthritis tend to have a higher number of risk factorsTrusted Source for cardiovascular disease than the general population, including increased BMI, triglycerides, and C-reactive protein.

Gout

Gout is a rheumatic disease that happens when uric acid crystals, or monosodium urate, form in body tissues and fluids. It happens when the body produces too much uric acid or does not excrete enough uric acid.

Gout causes agonizing pain in the joint, with the area becoming red, hot and swollen.

Acute gout normally appears as a severely red, hot, and swollen joint and severe pain.

Risk factors include:

• overweight or obesity

- hypertension

- alcohol intake

- use of diuretics

- a diet rich in meat and seafood

- some common medicines

- poor kidney function

Long periods of remission are possible, followed by flares lasting from days to weeks. Sometimes it can be chronic. Recurrent attacks of acute gout can lead to a degenerative form of chronic arthritis called gouty arthritis.

Sjögren's syndrome

Sjögren's syndrome is an autoimmune disorder that sometimes occurs alongside

RA and SLE. It involves the destruction of glands that produce tears and saliva. This causes dryness in the mouth and eyes and in other areas that usually need moisture, such as the nose, throat, and skin.

It can also affect the joints, lungs, kidneys, blood vessels, digestive organs, and nerves.

Sjögren's syndrome typically affects in adults aged 40 to 50 years, and especially women.

According to a study in Clinical and Experimental Rheumatology, in 40 to 50 percentTrusted Source of people with primary Sjögren's syndrome, the condition affects tissues other than the glands.

It could affect the lungs, liver, or kidneys, or it could lead to skin vasculitis, peripheral neuropathy, glomerulonephritis, and low levels of a substance known as C4. These all indicate a link between Sjögren's and the immune system.

If these tissues are affected, there is a high risk of developing non-Hodgkin's lymphoma.

Scleroderma

Scleroderma refers to a group of diseases that affect connective tissue in the body. The person will have patches of hard, dry skin. Some types can affect the internal organs and small arteries.

Scar-like tissue builds up in the skin and causes damage.

The cause is currently unknown. It often affects people between the ages of 30 to 50 years, and it may occur with other autoimmune diseases, such as lupus.

Scleroderma affects individuals differently. The complications include skin problems, weakness in the heart, lung damage, gastrointestinal problems, and kidney failure.

Systemic lupus erythematosus (SLE)

SLE, commonly known as lupus, is an autoimmune disease where the immune system produces antibodies to cells within the body leading toTrusted Source widespread inflammation and tissue damage. The disease is characterized by periods of illness and remissions.

It can appear at any age, but onset is most likelyTrusted Source is between the ages of 15 and 45 years. For every one man who gets lupus, between 4 and 12 women will do so.

Lupus can affect the joints, skin, brain, lungs, kidneys, blood vessels, and other tissues. Symptoms include fatigue, pain or swelling in joints, skin rashes, and fevers.

The cause remains unclear, but it could be linked to genetic, environmental, and hormonal factors.

NATURAL REMEDIES
A healthful, balanced diet with appropriate exercise, avoiding smoking, and not drinking excess alcohol can help people with arthritis maintain their overall health.

Diet

There is no specific diet that treats arthritis, but some types of food may help reduce inflammation.

The following foods, found in a Mediterranean diet, can provide many nutrients that are good for joint health:

• fish

• nuts and seeds

• fruits and vegetables

• beans

• olive oil

• whole grains

Foods to avoid

There are some foods that people with arthritis may want to avoid.

Nightshade vegetables, such as tomatoes, contain a chemical called solanine that some studies have linked with arthritis pain. Research findings are mixed when it comes to these vegetables, but some people have reported a reduction in arthritis symptoms when avoiding nightshade vegetables.

Self-management

Self-management of arthritis symptoms is also important.

Key strategies include:

• staying physically active

• achieving and maintaining a healthy weight

• getting regular check-ups with the doctor

• protecting joints from unnecessary stress

Seven habits that can help a person with arthritis to manage their condition are:

1. Being organized: keep track of symptoms, pain levels, medications, and possible side effects for consultations with your doctor.

2. Managing pain and fatigue: a medication regimen can be combined with non-medical pain management. Learning to manage fatigue is key to living comfortably with arthritis.

3. Staying active: exercise is beneficial for managing arthritis and overall health.

4. Balancing activity with rest: in addition to remaining active, rest is equally important when your disease is active.

5. Eating a healthful diet: a balanced diet can help you achieve a healthy weight and control inflammation. Avoid refined, processed foods and pro-inflammatory animal-derived foods and choose whole plant foods that are high in antioxidants and that have anti-inflammatory properties.

6. Improving sleep: poor sleep can aggravate arthritis pain and fatigue. Take steps to improve sleep hygiene so you find it easier to fall asleep and stay asleep. Avoid caffeine and strenuous exercise in

the evenings and restrict screen-time just before sleeping.

7. Caring for joints: tips for protecting joints include using the stronger, larger joints as levers when opening doors, using several joints to spread the weight of an object such as using a backpack and gripping as loosely as possible by using padded handles.

Do not sit in the same position for long periods. Take regular breaks to keep mobile.

Physical therapies

Doctors will often recommend a course of physical therapy to help patients with arthritis overcome some of the challenges and to reduce limitations on mobility.

• Warm water therapy: exercises in a warm-water pool. The water supports weight and puts less pressure on the muscles and joints

• Physical therapy: specific exercises tailored to the condition and individual needs, sometimes combined with pain-relieving treatments such as ice or hot packs and massage

• Occupational therapy: practical advice on managing everyday tasks, choosing specialized aids and equipment, protecting the joints from further damage and managing fatigue

Research suggests that although individuals with arthritis may experience short-term increases in pain when first beginning exercise, continued physical activity can be an effective way to reduce symptomsTrusted Source long-term.

People with arthritis can participate in joint-friendly physical activity on their own or with friends. As many people with arthritis have another condition, such as heart disease, it is important to choose appropriate activities.

Joint-friendly physical activities that are appropriate for adults with arthritis and heart disease include:

• walking

• swimming

• cycling

A health care professional can help you find ways to live a healthful lifestyle and have a better quality of life.

Natural therapies

A number of natural remedies have been suggested for different types of arthritis.

According to the organization Versus Arthritis, based in the United Kingdom (U.K.), some research has supported the use of devil's claw, rosehip, and Boswellia, from the frankincense tree. Devil's claw and Boswellia supplements can be purchased online.

There is some evidenceTrusted Source that turmeric may help, but more studies are needed to confirm their effectiveness.

Various other herbs and spices have been recommended for RA, but again, more research is needed. They include turmeric, garlic, ginger, black pepper, and green tea.

Many of these herbs and spices are available to purchase online in supplement form, including turmeric, ginger, and garlic.

Anyone who is considering using natural remedies for any type of arthritis should speak to a doctor first.

Early signs

The symptoms of arthritis that appear and how they appear vary widely, depending on the type.

Warning signs of arthritis include pain, swelling, stiffness and difficulty moving a joint.

They can develop gradually or suddenly. As arthritis is most often a chronic disease, symptoms may come and go, or persist over time.

However, anyone who experiences any of the following four key warning signs should see a doctor.

1. Pain: Pain from arthritis can be constant, or it may come and go. It may affect only one part, or be felt in many parts of the body

2. Swelling: In some types of arthritis the skin over the affected joint becomes red and swollen and feels warm to the touch

3. Stiffness. Stiffness is a typical symptom. With some types, this is most likely upon waking up in the morning, after sitting at a desk, or after sitting in a car for a long time. With other types, stiffness may occur after exercise, or it may be persistent.

4. Difficulty moving a joint: If moving a joint or getting up from a chair is hard or painful, this could indicate arthritis or another joint problem.

Rheumatoid arthritis

RA is a systemic disease, so it usually affects the joints on both sides of the body equally. The joints of the wrists, fingers, knees, feet and ankles are the most commonly affected.

Joint symptoms may include:

• morning stiffness, lasting more than 1 hour

• pain, often in the same joints on both sides of the body

• loss of range of motion of joints, possibly with deformity

Other symptoms include:

• chest pain when breathing in, due to pleurisy

• dry eyes and mouth, if Sjögren's syndrome is present

• eye burning, itching, and discharge

• nodules under the skin, usually a sign of more severe disease

• numbness, tingling, or burning in the hands and feet

• sleep difficulties

Osteoarthritis

Osteoarthritis is usually a result of wear and tear on the joints. It will affect joints that have been overworked more than others. People with osteoarthritis may experience the following symptoms:

• pain and stiffness in the joints

• pain that becomes worse after exercise or pressure on the joint

• rubbing, grating, or crackling sound when a joint is moved

• morning stiffness

• pain that causes sleep disturbances

Some people may have changes linked to osteoarthritis that show up in an x-ray, but they do not experience symptoms.

Osteoarthritis typically affects some joints more than others, such as the left or right knee, shoulder or wrist.

Childhood arthritis

Symptoms of childhood arthritis include:
• a joint that is swollen, red, or warm

• a joint that is stiff or limited in movement

• limping or difficulty using an arm or leg

• a sudden high fever that may come and go

• a rash on the trunk and extremities that comes and goes with the fever

• symptoms throughout the body, such as pale skin, swollen lymph glands

• generally appearing unwell

Juvenile RA can also cause eye problems including uveitis, iridocyclitis, or iritis. If eye symptoms do occur they can include:

• red eyes

• eye pain, especially when looking at light

• vision changes.

Septic arthritis

Symptoms of septic arthritis occur rapidly.

There is often:

• fever

• intense joint pain that becomes more severe with movement

• joint swelling in one joint

Symptoms in newborns or infants include:

• crying when the infected joint is moved

• fever

• inability to move the limb with the infected joint

• irritability

Symptoms in children and adults include:

• inability to move the limb with the infected joint

• intense joint pain, swelling, and redness

• fever.

Chills sometimes occur but are an uncommon symptom.

Fibromyalgia

Fibromyalgia may trigger the following Trusted Source symptoms:

Fibromyalgia has many symptoms that tend to vary from person to person. The main symptom is widespread pain.

• widespread pain, often with specific tender points

• sleep disturbance

• fatigue

• psychological stress

• morning stiffness

• tingling or numbness in hands and feet

• headaches, including migraines

• irritable bowel syndrome

• problems with thinking and memory, sometimes called "fibro fog"

• Painful menstrual periods and other pain syndromes

Psoriatic arthritis

Symptoms of psoriatic arthritis may be mild and involve only a few joints such as the end of the fingers or toes.

Severe psoriatic arthritis can affect multiple joints, including the spine. Spinal symptoms are usually felt in the lower spine and sacrum. These consist of stiffness, burning, and pain.

People with psoriatic arthritis often have the skin and nail changes of psoriasis, and the skin gets worse at the same time as the arthritis.

Gout

Symptoms of gout involve:

• pain and swelling, often in the big toe, knee, or ankle joints

• sudden pain, often during the night, which may be throbbing, crushing, or excruciating

• warm and tender joints that appear red and swollen

• fever sometimes occurs

After having gout for many years, a person can develop tophi. Tophi are lumps below the skin, typically around the joints or apparent on fingertips and ears. Multiple, small tophi may develop, or a large white lump. This can cause deformation and stretching of the skin.

Sometimes, tophi burst and drain spontaneously, oozing a white, chalky substance. Tophi that are beginning to break through the skin can lead to infection or osteomyelitis. Some patients will need urgent surgery to drain the tophus.

Sjögren's syndrome

Symptoms of Sjögren's syndrome include:

• dry and itchy eyes, and a feeling that something is in the eye

- dry mouth

- difficulty swallowing or eating

- loss of sense of taste

- problems speaking

- thick or stringy saliva

- mouth sores or pain

- hoarseness

- fatigue

- fever

- change in color of hands or feet

- joint pain or joint swelling

- swollen glands

Scleroderma

Symptoms of scleroderma may include:

• fingers or toes that turn blue or white in response to cold temperatures, known as Raynaud's phenomenon

• hair loss

• skin that becomes darker or lighter than normal

• stiffness and tightness of skin on the fingers, hands, forearm, and face

• small white lumps beneath the skin that sometimes ooze a white substance that looks like toothpaste

• sores or ulcers on the fingertips or toes

• tight and mask-like skin on the face

• numbness and pain in the feet

• pain, stiffness, and swelling of the wrist, fingers, and other joints

• dry cough, shortness of breath, and wheezing

• gastrointestinal problems, such as bloating after meals, constipation, and diarrhea

• difficulty swallowing

• esophageal reflux or heartburn

Systemic lupus erythematosus (SLE)

The most common signs of SLE, or lupus, are:

• red rash or color change on the face, often in the shape of a butterfly across the nose and cheeks

• painful or swollen joints

• unexplained fever

• chest pain when breathing deeply

• swollen glands

• extreme fatigue

• unusual hair loss

• pale or purple fingers or toes from cold or stress

• sensitivity to the sun

• low blood count

• depression, trouble thinking or memory problems.

Other signs are mouth sores, unexplained seizures, hallucinations, repeated miscarriages, and unexplained kidney problems.

CBD Guidance for Adults with Arthritis

The Issue

The Arthritis Foundation is aware of the growing popularity and availability of CBD-based products. Industry reports show that people with arthritis are among the top buyers, and pain is the leading reason for purchase. Our July 2019 survey of 2,600 people with arthritis shows significant use of and interest in CBD(cannabidiol).* Earlier surveys have shown repeatedly that pain is the most burdensome arthritis symptom.

The Arthritis Foundation Position

As the largest organization representing the voice and needs of people with arthritis, the Arthritis Foundation has always welcomed new treatment options because no single drug, supplement or therapy works for everyone. We believe patients should be empowered to find safe management strategies that are appropriate for them. The more options available, the likelier it is that more people will benefit.

We are intrigued by the potential of CBD to help people find pain relief and are on record urging the FDA to expedite the study and regulation of these products. While currently there is limited scientific evidence about CBD's ability to help ease arthritis symptoms, and no universal quality standards or regulations exist, we have listened to our constituents and consulted with leading experts to develop these general recommendations for adults who are interested in trying CBD.

• CBD may help with arthritis-related symptoms, such as pain, insomnia and anxiety, but there have been no rigorous clinical studies in people with arthritis to confirm this.

• While no major safety issues have been found with CBD when taken in moderate doses, potential drug interactions have been identified.

• CBD should never be used to replace disease-modifying drugs that help prevent permanent joint damage in inflammatory types of arthritis.

• CBD use should be discussed with your doctor in advance, with follow-up evaluations every three months or so, as would be done for any new treatment.

• There are no established clinical guidelines to inform usage. Experts recommend starting with a low dose, and if relief is inadequate, increase in small increments weekly.

• Buy from a reputable company that has each batch tested for purity, potency and safety by an independent laboratory and provides a certificate of analysis.

What is CBD? CBD, short for cannabidiol, is an active compound found in the cannabis plant. CBD is not intoxicating but may cause some drowsiness. The CBD in most products is extracted from hemp, a variety of cannabis that has only traces (up to 0.3%) of THC, the active compound that gets people high.

Does CBD work for arthritis? Animal studies have suggested that CBD has pain-relieving and anti-inflammatory properties, but these effects have not been validated in quality studies in humans. Anecdotally, some people with arthritis who have tried CBD, but not all, report noticeable pain relief, sleep improvement and/or anxiety reduction.

Is CBD safe to use? Research evaluating the safety of CBD is underway. At this point very little is known. So far, no serious safety concerns have been associated with moderate doses. CBD is thought to have the potential to interact with some drugs commonly taken by people with arthritis. Talk to your doctor before trying CBD if you take any of the following: corticosteroids (such as prednisone), tofacitinib (Xeljanz), naproxen (Aleve), celecoxib (Celebrex), tramadol (Ultram), certain antidepressants, including amitriptyline (Elavil), citalopram (Celexa), fluoxetine (Prozac), mirtazapine (Remeron), paroxetine (Paxil), sertraline (Zoloft), and certain medications for fibromyalgia, including gabapentin (Neurontin) and pregabalin (Lyrica).

Should I give CBD a try? Without quality clinical studies on CBD and arthritis, doctors have not been able to say who might benefit from CBD, at what dose and in which form, who likely won't benefit and who should avoid it. Still, there is agreement on several points:

• CBD is not a substitute for disease-modifying treatment for inflammatory arthritis.

• Patients who are interested in trying CBD should first talk to the health care provider who treats their arthritis before trying CBD. Together, they can review what has worked or not worked in the past, whether there are other options to try first, how to do a trial run, what to watch for and when to return for a follow-up visit to evaluate the results. Keep a symptom and dose diary to track effects.

• Quality CBD products can be expensive, especially when used for prolonged periods. To avoid wasting money, be completely sure that the product is truly having a positive effect on symptoms.

What type of product should I consider? CBD-based products can be taken orally, applied to the skin or inhaled. There are pros and cons for each.

By mouth. CBD that is swallowed, whether in capsules, food or liquid, is absorbed through the digestive tract. Absorption is slow and dosing is tricky due to the delayed onset of effect (one to two hours), unknown effects of stomach acids, recent meals and other factors.

Capsules can work for daily use after a safe, effective capsule dose has been established. Experts discourage taking CBD via edibles, like gummies and cookies, because dosing is unreliable, and they are appealing to children but do not come in childproof containers. Like any medicine, edibles should be secured out of sight and reach of children.

CBD can also be absorbed directly into the bloodstream by holding liquid from a spray or tincture (a liquid dosed by a dropper) under the tongue (sublingual) for 60 to 120 seconds. The taste may not be pleasant. Effects may be felt within 15 to 45 minutes.

On the skin. Topical products, like lotions and balms, are applied to the skin over a painful joint. Whether these products deliver CBD below the skin is unknown. Topical products may also include common over-the-counter ingredients such as menthol, capsaicin or camphor, making it difficult to determine if a positive effect is due to the CBD or another ingredient.

Inhaled. CBD can be inhaled via a vaporizing, or vape, pen. However, inhalation of vapor oils and chemical byproducts carry unknown risks, particularly for people with inflammatory arthritis. For this reason and because the

Centers for Disease Control and Prevention is investigating vaping in association with widespread hospitalizations and deaths from severe pulmonary disease, vaping is not recommended.

How much CBD you should use

While there are no established clinical guidelines, the medical experts consulted by the Arthritis Foundation recommend the following for adults:

• When preparing to take a liquid form, be aware that the CBD extract is mixed with a carrier oil, so there are two measures to know: the amount of the liquid product to take (the dose) and the amount of CBD in each dose.

• Go low and slow. Start with just a few milligrams of CBD in sublingual form twice a day. If relief is inadequate after one week, increase the dose by that same amount. If needed, go up in small increments over several weeks. If you find relief, continue taking that dose twice daily to maintain a stable level of CBD in the blood.

• If CBD alone doesn't work and you are in a state where medical or recreational marijuana is legal, talk to your doctor about taking CBD with a very low-dose THC product. Be aware that THC, even at low levels, may get you high, creating cognitive, motor and balance issues. Try THC-containing products at home or at night first, so you can sleep off any unwanted effects.

• After several weeks, if you don't find relief with CBD alone or with a combination of CBD and very low THC, CBD may not be right for you.

• If you experience any unwanted side effects when using a CBD product, immediately discontinue use and inform your doctor.

www.ingramcontent.com/pod-product-compliance
Lightning Source LLC
Chambersburg PA
CBHW061728250726
48657CB00002B/820